# Steps To take Before Starting A Weight Loss Program

By:

# DR. A. HAKEEM, PH.D., N.C., BIO-C.P.

Copyright © 2015 by: Dr. A. Hakeem

All Rights Reserved.

Published in the USA by The Center for Natural Living, Inc.

5603 W. Friendly Ave. Suite B, Greensboro, NC. 27410

Email: drhakeem1@gmail.com

Fax: (336) 316-0171

Website: www.thecenterfornaturalliving.com

Always consult a physician before starting any diet plan.

This book offers health, fitness and nutritional information and is designed for educational purposes only. Do not disregard, avoid or delay obtaining medical or health related advice from your health-care professional because of something you may have read in this book. You should not rely on this information as a substitute for, nor does it replace, professional medical advice, diagnosis, or treatment.

# Congratulations

You have just taken a giant step forward in taking responsibility for your own health.

The weight loss and removal of toxins from your body is a powerful tool that will help you to look and feel your best.

# Table of Contents

# CHAPTER 1

# Affirmations, Goals, and Your Plans

What if an immensely powerful tool were available for you to use any time you wanted? There is such a tool, and it comes from within YOU.

Where do you start? The aligning of one's body, mind, and spirit is routinely done through the use of Affirmations. To affirm means "to state as a fact; assert strongly and publicly."

For example, "The president affirmed the country's commitment to peace." Synonyms for affirm include declare, state, assert, proclaim, pronounce, avow, attest, swear, guarantee, and pledge. We make affirmations because they are important to keep us on task and to prevent our wandering off course. You can adopt and use these examples of affirmations as your own as you pursue your goal of healthier living.

Affirmation 1: I have transformed my health and lifestyle, and I am healthier than I have been in years.

Affirmation 2: I am transforming my lifestyle to a healthier and more complete way of living through my spirit, mind, and body.

Affirmation 3: I am winning at losing weight and regaining my health in ways I never expected. I have never felt better or more connected spiritually, physically, and mentally.

Feel free to develop your own affirmation that motivates you to stay on track and to win. Dive in! You can do it, and you will soon be swimming in goals and affirmations.

Remember: Goals without plans = Failure.

You must have a series of plans and objectives that move progressively toward a goal. Setting goals is only the first step of the process. To be successful in achieving your goal, you need a plan.

**To Be Successful at Weight Loss You must:**

- Have the desire
- Be determined
- Be committed to being healthy
- Be courageous
- Make sacrifices
- Be patient
- Be strong
- Make preparations
- Ask for God's Holy Spirit
- Have a budget for your program

Without a detailed plan that supports your targets and goals, they remain wishful thinking. The steps you follow are what make achieving your goals possible. Ideas, preparation, knowledge, and wisdom are useless without a framework that is put into action.

Swear off all fried foods, processed foods, and wheat products. Remove all dairy products including milk, butter, and cheese. Have milk substitutes including rice, almond, oat, or soy milk. Remove bread from your life. Once grain is processed into some sort of bread, its nutritional value is destroyed.

If you can, shop at the local farmers market for your fresh produce.

The diet you have today,
may determine your health
in the future.

# CHAPTER 2

# Thin for Life

There is not one way that works for everyone to lose weight. One size does not fit all.

The eight keys to successful weight management are:

1) Believe that you will become thin for life. Ignore all those commonly held negative notions about weight management, such as "It's hard to lose weight after a certain age." You just have to know how.

2) Stop looking to others for answers. They do not have answers, but they will continue giving you advice if you keep asking. Do not tell others what you are doing if you want to remain on your program.

3) Find a Natural Health Coach or a skilled practitioner, and have him or her design a program individualized for you. I help with this daily.

4) Accept the food facts. Contrary to what advertisers may tell you, you cannot eat all you want. That is what got you into the condition you desire to change. Once you reach your optimal weight, to return to your old habits is diet suicide.

5)  Learn the art of positive self-speak. Never say anything about yourself that you do not intend to make "law." Negative thoughts and statements are debilitating and life-stealing. They stick to you like a magnet. All negative thoughts run counter to your weight management goals.

6)  Start a regular exercise program which is appropriate to your body type and physical limitations, and stick to it. Increase your favorite physical activity to help keep your weight off once you get to your goal.

7)  Learn to deal with life's problems in a constructive way, and remember stress is reduced by supporting your liver. *(More on this later.)* Get more out of life by taking time to enjoy it. Balance your life with work, hobbies, friendship, a strong religious foundation, and travel, and you will have a better chance of controlling your weight.

8)  Do not be in a hurry to lose weight. You should lose between two and three pounds a week.

**Breakfast:** Eat a good breakfast of fruit or smoothies. Guidelines for breakfast are described later in this chapter.

**Lunch:** Lunch should be eaten between 11 a.m. and 2 p.m. and should be your largest meal of the day. Lunch choices are described later in this chapter.

**Cut Out:** Fatty foods such as meats and meat products, mayonnaise, salad dressings, cheese, and dairy products. Processed sugars and sodas should also be removed from your diet.

Eat a variety of leafy greens, yellow vegetables, and root vegetables. Be sure to include fresh fruit, fresh unpasteurized juices, and whole grains in your meal plans.

Do not snack late at night or between meals.

Skip all desserts. They are mouth-pleasing treats that are torture for your health and body shape.

Do not drink coffee or any other caffeinated beverages.

**Dinner:** If eaten, it should not be eaten after 8 p.m. Lightly steamed and raw vegetables are best. You can add beans or yams *(no sugar)*, or have a Whey Protein Powder Shake. It is preferable not to have water while eating, but if you must, have hot water with lemon.

*Dinner, although popular, is one of the worst meals we can eat. Dinner is contrary to nature and the circadian rhythms which direct us and all life on the planet. Work to make dinner a social event where eating is not the focus.*

**After-Dinner Walk:** Whether you choose to eat dinner or not, take a nice walk in the early evening or after your dinner meal. Make your walk a social event.

If you need something comforting at bedtime, you can have herbal tea, such as red clover, green tea, spearmint tea, etc. but **no caffeine**.

Drink plenty of pure spring or reverse-osmosis filtered water, 80 to 120 ounces a day, or more as needed. Never drink distilled or alkaline water. They run contrary to our health, regardless of what you may have heard.

Do not drink water while eating your meals. It is guaranteed to slow your digestion.

**Enzymes:** Use digestive enzymes to aid digestion if you like. Whole raw fruit and vegetables are rich in them, so you really shouldn't need additional ones.

**Natural Iron:** Purchase a bottle of liquid chlorophyll, put a tablespoon in six ounces of water, and drink it down.

**Fasting:** Fasting is fully discussed in Chapter 14: Other Weight Loss Methods.

## Your Morning Routine

Upon waking, to help activate your immune system and to boost your metabolism, do the following:

Thoroughly scrape your tongue using a spoon or tongue scraper.

Brush your teeth.

Wash your face with warm, not hot, water, followed by a good splash of cold water.

Drink 10 ounces of room temperature water with ½ ounce of fresh squeezed organic citrus juice *(orange, lemon, lime, grapefruit, tangerine, or pomelo)* with two pinches of cayenne powder mixed into the water. Squeeze the juice yourself. Do not buy it already squeezed.

Take 8 minutes of deep, cleansing breaths.

Stretch your back and legs for 15 minutes.

Drink another 6 ounces of room temperature water and citrus juice prepared the same way as shown on previous page.

## Your Breakfast

Breakfast should consist of organic fruit that supports and activates your digestive tract. The fruits that do this best are the citrus fruits: oranges, tangerines, lemons, limes, grapefruit, pomelos, tangelos, and kumquats.

Ideally, a plate of a single fruit is preferable to mixed fruits. This method removes almost all stress from the digestive process.

If organic fruit is not available, it is better to eat non-organic fruit than not to eat fruit at all. strawberries, raspberries, blackberries, blueberries, kiwi, Granny Smith apples.

Every other day, you may substitute fresh organic pears, peaches, apples, or pineapple.

## Your Lunch

Lunch can consist of lightly steamed veggies or a salad consisting of red or green lettuce, tomato slices or wedges, celery, bell peppers, shredded carrots, basil or cilantro, and fennel, topped with an optional slice of steamed fish or baked organic chicken.

Salad dressing should consist of lemon juice or pureed apple or orange with a touch of ginger.

## Daily Snacks

Snacks are not meals. They are bits of sustenance which are excellent for calming appetite cravings.

You can eat grapes, orange wedges, cherry tomatoes, an apple wedge, two or three strawberries, ½ grapefruit, a wedge of pineapple, and/or a slice of seasonal watermelon.

## The No-Nos

During the first 45 days of your weight loss plan:

No nuts or seeds of any type.

No butters.
Absolutely NO dairy. No milk, cheese, butter, yogurt, ice cream, creamer, cream sauces, etc.

Do not eat store brought cream gravies and salad dressings. These are man-invented concoctions that stop weight loss by polluting the body. Replace the creams with rice, soy, almond, tofu, or oat milk.

Do not ever eat dry cereals of any type.

Do not consume caffeine from any source. This means no coffee, decaf, espresso, tea, yerba mate, soda, energy drinks, No-Doz, or chewing coffee beans.

No sugar or sweeteners of any type.

Do not drink carbonated beverages, soda, or seltzer. Replace with spring water, filtered water, or reverse osmosis water, or fresh-squeezed organic fruit juice.

No wheat or grains. Nature does not make sandwiches or cereal.

# CHAPTER 3

# Who Are You?

Most people want the answer to the question, "Am I obese, or am I just overweight?" Some general guidelines for determining your classification are as follows:

| Percentage Body Fat | Body Type |
|---|---|
| 2 – 8% | Excellent, highly athletic body type |
| 9 -12% | Very healthy, also potentially athletic |
| 13-17% | Good, but can be better |
| 18-20% | Normal, but on the fringes of being overweight |
| 21-23% | Overweight, teetering on obesity |
| 24% or Higher | Obese |

Generally speaking, if you can shake the body fat in your abdomen like jelly, then it is safe to say you are overweight or obese. If you cannot see your beltline because your belly is in the way, you are definitely obese.

With work, your body can become one that you will be proud to show off in public.

"Change is never easy,
you fight to hold on
and you fight to let go."

# CHAPTER 4

# It's Time For A Change

To improve your health by losing weight, you will need to make a change. Food habits are not easy to change, because most people have well-established cooking and social habits.

While we are getting along well in life, we rarely consider the connection between food and our health. We often find it difficult to recognize the relationship between the food we eat and what happens to our hair, nails, skin, and eyes, but there is definitely a relationship here.

In the United States, we have never had training about this connection. Why not? To put it simply, in the western illness-based economy, we are all worth more sick than healthy. We do not know that our bloodstream depends on what we eat. We don't know that what we eat today will walk and talk tomorrow. We don't know that what we consume actually becomes the cells, bones, and organs of our body. This is why, unless we change our faulty ways of eating, we can never expect a permanent turn for the better in our health.

A simple, yet neglected, question is, "How long do you want to live?" Yes, we are all going to die some day, so the next question is, "Should you die in a nursing home with oatmeal dribbling down your chin, playing bingo with people you can not recall from one day to the next?" Fifty percent of those who live until age 65 will spend the final years of their lives in misery in a nursing home.

Will you be one of the 50% who wait for symptoms to engulf you and dictate the conditions you experience for the rest of your life? If you wait too long, that is exactly what will happen. Can you control your aging so that stroke, cancer, dementia, arthritis, and diapers are not part of your future? Is it possible to feel 25 until the day you die?

Those who understand the role of food and personal detoxification say they feel far younger than their years. The time to make changes is now.

# CHAPTER 5

# Apple or Pear?

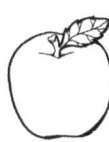 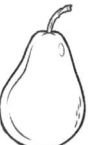

Your physical shape speaks volumes about your personal health risks. Ayurveda, a centuries-old holistic approach to health from the Vedic area of India, classifies body shape and density as Pitta, Kapha, and Vata. In a later chapter, you will be instructed in how to use these body types to pick the kind of exercise that will be best for you.

For every decade of adulthood, most people gain weight. On average, we gain between 2.5 and 7.5 pounds a year, unless we are determined not to allow it to happen.

Where your weight settles determines another kind of classification based on body shape. If your weight sinks to your buttocks, hips, and thighs, you have a "pear" shape. If you carry fat in and around your abdominal organs, with a "pot belly" or "spare tire," you have an "apple" shape, which is associated with increased likelihood of current and future disease.

Diabetes is a frequent result of body distortion caused by diet. Coronary artery disease, stroke, high blood pressure, and even cancer are linked to being overweight or, now more commonly, obese.

"Apples," because of excess fat in the abdomen, that is likely to release or break down causing it to enter the blood stream. Regardless of their weight once in the blood, liquefied lipids can clog the arteries *(atherosclerosis)*.

Over-eating, drinking alcohol in excess, and not getting enough – or any – exercise, also creates "apples and pears."

In conjunction with body shape, waist measurement is useful in determining where you are carrying too much weight. Find the highest point on each hipbone, and measure around your waist just above these points. A measurement exceeding 40 inches for men or 35 inches for women indicates significantly increased risk of disease. In general, the bigger your waist gets, the greater your health risks.

CHAPTER 6

# What Causes Weight Gain?

Excess starchy foods, breads, refined sugar, pasta, rice, sucrose, lactose, maltose, alcohol, and parasites form the basis of weight gain. These ten items can lead to poor digestion – which some call food allergies – that lead to candidiasis *(overgrowth of Candida yeast)* and bloating, flatulence, and weight gain. When these conditions persist, underactive thyroid gland, hypoglycemia, inflammation, and other problems can result. Inflammation is our worst enemy, causing the body to start gaining weight.

Processed, high-glycemic carbohydrates such as potato chips, corn chips, rice cakes, corn cakes, cookies, pretzels, crackers, candy, and starchy foods cause a spike in blood sugar that can last hours, resulting in elevated insulin production from the pancreas. If insulin is released too quickly, it leads to a drop in blood sugar and a repeat of the whole cycle. The more we eat, the hungrier we feel until we are bloated, swollen, and miserable. Many people experience this vicious cycle several times a day, leading directly to rapid weight gain.

Toxic foods convert to sugar in the blood stream, resulting in insulin release, which causes the body to store fat. Cooking food at temperatures over 105 degrees kills enzymes, leaving us with a mixture that offers vitamins but no food enzymes.

In addition, emotional upset may cause us to start eating again, for the wrong reasons. Eating too late at night is another killer, interrupting body repair cycles and ruining sleep for many. The last meal of the day should be eaten at least four hours before bed time. Many people skip dinner completely and report positive results.

Hormone imbalance may seem mysterious to many people, but it finds its beginnings in our diet choices, and we gain weight in response. Females 35 years old or older and men 40 years old or older are the most susceptible to hormonal weight gain. Yet, everyone is capable of adopting a collection of habits that will result in body-wide inflammation and weight gain. To assure good health, you must cultivate the habits that suppress inflammation and protect your body from hormonal imbalance.

In summary, insulin sensitivity, underactive thyroid, poor digestion, too little exercise, toxin loading, nutritional deficiencies, stress, and inadequate rest all lead to acidosis in the body and inflammation. Eating processed foods and/or not drinking enough water can lead to tissue swelling and to kidney/adrenal gland fatigue, and stress, finally resulting in weight gain.

### Why Are So Many Overweight?

For decades a debate has gone on about the best way to lose weight. Even aggressive "diets" have failed to achieve significant fat loss. The problem has been our dancing around the underlying factors that cause excess body fat.

Researchers have identified specific biological mechanisms that are believed to cause aging and weight gain, no matter how little we eat. In order to lose weight, we need a direct assault. Are you ready to gain control over your body's command signals that are critical to maintaining a healthy body weight?

## Leptin Resistance

Leptin is a hormone that tells the brain that we have consumed enough calories and we can stop eating. Leptin induces a process which breaks down fat stored in cells. As we age, our cells, including the appetite control center in our brain, become "leptin resistant." This means that leptin is unable to regulate body weight effectively.

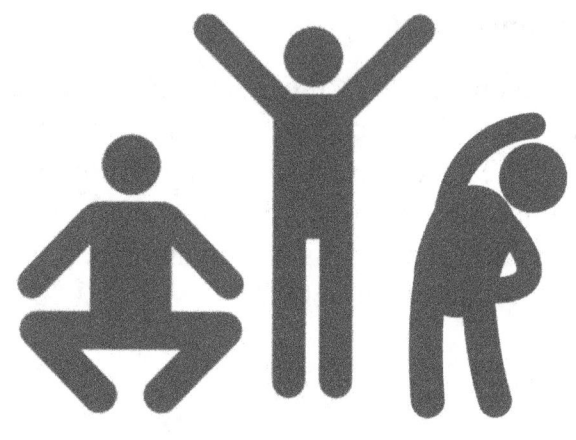

Are You Ready?

CHAPTER 7

# Before You Start

**Be sure your body is ready to execute your plans.**

Before you become active in your weight loss endeavor, you will need to see a doctor for a full check up to be sure your body is able to support you in supporting it. Trying to lose weight while dealing with a major illness is not advisable.

The first thing to do is to find a physician who is interested in preventive as well as therapeutic medicine. You should have no difficulty discussing your interests and health objectives with your doctor. If your current doctor's personality meshes with yours, you can stay with him or her. If the two of you are compatible, you will have a weight loss partner who will be as excited about your progress as you are. If not, find a holistic practitioner such as a naturopath, homeopath, chiropractor, etc. who relates well to you and whom you would like to accompany you on your journey.

**Get started the right way.**

Once you have chosen your practitioner, schedule a full physical, and request a blood panel or weight loss blood panel. These tests will allow you to determine whether there are any underlying health issues that should be addressed before you start.

Let your doctor tell you how much exercise and weight training is appropriate for you.

Once you have your doctor's lab work, and blood panel, be sure to get a copy for your records. Then get started, and have a great weight loss experience.

CHAPTER 8

# Body Types and Exercise

As noted in Chapter 4, the Ayurvedic body types are Vata, Pitta, and Kapha. By determining your body type, you can choose exercises which are appropriate for you.

**Vata – Small Frame**

If you have a small frame, you are a Vata. The best exercises for this type of body frame are medium-paced walks, stretches, Tai Chi, and yoga stretching.

**Pitta – Medium Frame**

The Pitta, medium framed body type, needs cooling exercises like swimming, water aerobics, and nature walks or walking in the cool of the evening or early in the morning at sunrise.

**Kapha – Large Frame**

Generally Kapha body types are ones who have good stamina, but are heavy and slow, making them lethargic. This group should do aerobic exercises, jogging, running, or aerobic sports such as tennis, soccer, or basketball five to six times a week.

## All Body Types

Some exercises such as bicycling, walking, swimming, and dancing are balancing for all body types. Select the exercise you feel best with, because, in the end, exercise not done is a waste that will keep your waist from shrinking.

# CHAPTER 9

# Time to Shop
# Time to Get Busy

When it comes to a successful weight loss program, keep in mind that it is a treasure hunt and a supply hunt.

**What you will need:**

A full-length mirror. *(It is hard to control what you cannot see)*
A good pair of walking shoes.
A good blender.
A good juicer.

Clean your refrigerator of all junk and processed food. Eliminate all wheat and gluten from your house and your life.

Develop a regular exercise program of 45 minutes a day, four days a week. Develop a strength training program for 20 minutes a day, four days a week.

Use digestive enzymes with each of your meals, or eat an orange after every meal. Citrus is better than digestive enzymes at $\frac{1}{4}$ the cost.

Purchase all of the items and products you need to start your weight loss program before you start your journey.

You will need to do a whole body purification program for 15 weeks twice a year. I personally did eight months of purification when I started my weight loss program.

## Spring Rejuvenation

Many people think body purification is seasonal. This assumes that we are toxic only at certain times of the year. I assure you that toxicity is a 24/7, 365-days-a-year condition.

The most dangerous toxins are the ones the unnatural, man-made toxins that plague us all. Chemical warfare was banned after World War I because the effects were inhumane. Based on the results, big business has, for the past 75 years, continued to ignore the danger. In a more subtle way, our food, air, water, home and office appliances and furnishings, cleaning agents, solvents, fragrances, pesticides, and more contaminate us with such an intensity of toxins, that we are robbed of our vitality.

Inner cleansing or detoxification is a process of removing dead cells and waste (or toxins) from fatty tissue throughout the body. Over time, waste matter builds up in the body due to diet, environment, and pollutants we pick up from our cleaning and personal items such as antiperspirants. Everyday activities – like eating – produce more problems than most people can deal with comfortably. A poor diet is so hard to digest that it accumulates in the digestive tract like bricks and begins to putrefy. By the time the liver receives any of it, we are lucky to get any nutrients at all. This condition causes constipation, leaky gut syndrome, polyps, hemorrhoids, and other unpleasant results.

Poor digestion causes decreased levels of energy, circulation, and oxygen in the body. Getting these internal blockages and poisons out of the body is the first and most vital step in any health or beauty enhancement program.

## Who Should Not Do Inner Cleansing?

- If you are pregnant or nursing, do not do any inner cleansing, as you can pass the moving toxins on to your baby.

- If your doctor tells you not to engage in such a program, follow his or her directions.

## Reasons for Doing an Inner Cleanse

| | |
|---|---|
| Prevent disease | Increase productivity |
| Reduce symptoms | Clearer skin |
| Treat disease | Enjoy greater relaxation |
| Feel more attuned | Slow aging |
| Cleanse the body | Feel more energetic |
| Improve mental clarity | Improve flexibility |
| Rest the organs | Enhance consciousness |
| Be more organized | Improve fertility |
| Purification | Relationship focus |
| Enhance creativity | Enhance the senses |
| Rejuvenation | Greater emotional balance |
| Be more motivated | Improve sleep |
| Weight loss | Spiritual awareness |

Ideals, preparation, knowledge
and wisdom are useless....
Without Action.

# CHAPTER 10

# Extra-Large Fat Cells and The Cost Of Obesity

Adult-onset weight gain is characterized by the enlargement of existing adipocytes *(fat cells)* that store too much fat. The size of a fat cell is controlled by gene transcription factors. Fat cell size is closely related with adiponectin expression in the large fat cells. In addition, gene transcription factors help regulate adiponectin, the crucial hormone for supporting insulin sensitivity.

**Excess Activity of Fat Converting Enzyme**

An enzyme called glycerol-3-phosphate dehydrogenase is critical for synthesizing fatty acids in our bodies. Suppressing this enzyme helps reduce the amount of glucose *(sugar)* in the bloodstream being converted to fatty acids.

Weight loss plans including diet modification, professional supplements, hormones, or drugs usually function through a single mechanism. Adipocytes, on the other hand, possess numerous means to ensure their survival

Overweight and obesity are quite simply an excess of body fat. Anyone who is 20% above the norm for his/her age, body size, and height is considered overweight. Those who are over-weight for an extended time are more likely to experience kidney problems, liver damage, heart disease, diabetes, high blood pressure, gallbladder disease, arthritis, and certain cancers. The physical indicators also include high cholesterol, prostate cancer in men, breast cancer in women, fibromyalgia, and hyperinsulinemia and insulin resistance in either sex. When psychological problems and complications during pregnancy are factored in, we have the makings for ill health and escalating weight.

Some additional causes of obesity and weight gain include gallbladder malfunction, malnutrition, emotional tension, boredom, habits, and lust for food. Overweight and obesity have been linked to food sensitivity and allergies. Changing your food selection habits is a prime factor in whether you lose weight or become more overweight.

According to the Mayo Clinic, 63% of Americans are overweight or obese. Statistics indicate that 300,000 deaths a year are directly linked to obesity. It is not that people are not trying to trim, tuck, and tone. Although Americans spend over $34 billion a year on weight-loss products and services, few get good results. Based on the amount of money we spend on health care, Americans should be the leanest, healthiest people on Earth, but the numbers keep moving in the other direction. We are fighting the "battle of the bulge," but we are losing famously.

### The Cost of Obesity

Obesity is tied to an advanced risk of colorectal disease and increased likelihood of infection after colon surgery. According to a new study, obese patients are at significantly increased risk for surgical site infection after bowel surgery. The study included 7,020 patients, 1,243 of whom were obese, all between the ages of 18 and 64, who had total colon removal (colectomy) for colon cancer or partial removal for diverticulitis or inflammatory bowel disease between 2002 and 2008. The overall rate of surgical site infection was 10.3%, but the rate for obese patients was far higher. Even after adjusting for other factors, the obese patients were 60% more likely to develop surgical site infection than non-obese patients.

The average cost of colectomy for all patients was $16,399, but higher for obese patients. If a surgical site infection developed, the total cost jumped to $31,933 per affected patient. The convalescence or recovery time for patients without infection was 8.1 days compared to 9.5 days for patients with infections. Hospital readmissions among non-obese patients were 6.8% but 27.8% among obese patients.

"We concluded that patients undergoing colorectal surgery who develop [surgical site infections], many of whom are obese, tax the healthcare system." -*Surgical Site Infections and Cost in Obese Patients Undergoing Colorectal Surgery, Dr. Elizabeth C. Wick and colleagues, Johns Hopkins School of Medicine in Baltimore.*

Incentive programs which reward surgeons for keeping costs down and improving patient outcomes should take into account that obese people inflate surgical costs just by being obese. -*Surgical data pulled from Archives of Surgery.*

The risk of disease and complications of that disease start with and are increased by being obese. Obesity adds a nearly incalculable challenge to the lives of those who do not take control of their weight.

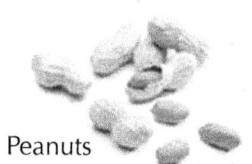

Peanuts

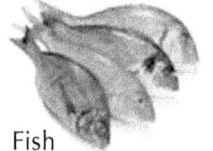

Fish

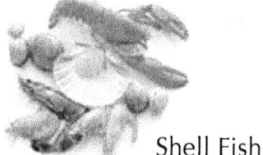

Shell Fish

# Possible Allergens

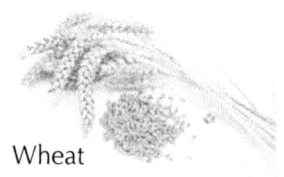

Wheat

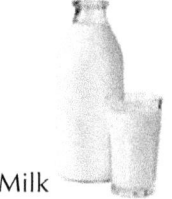

Milk

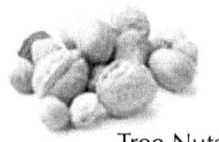

Tree Nuts

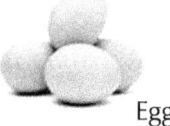

Eggs

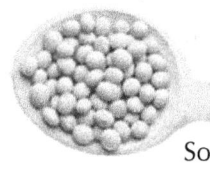

Soy

CHAPTER 11

# Food and Allergies

Every known food may at times cause some allergic reaction. Thus, the foods used in an "Elimination Diet" may cause allergies in some individuals, and a few of the foods are listed among those most likely to cause allergic reactions. However, the incidence of reaction to these foods is generally low, and they are widely used in making test diets. By keeping your own food journal, you will soon know your "problem foods." We all have certain foods that must be eliminated from our diets. If you have a repeated negative reaction after eating a particular food, it is reasonable to assume that you have an allergy to that food.

Some of the reactions that happen quickly upon exposure to allergens are: watery eyes, sneezing, coughing, stuffy nose, headache, feeling bloated, increased heart rate, dizziness, nasal drip, puffy bags under the eyes, worsening mood, chest pains, diarrhea, extreme thirst, tiredness, a sudden burst of energy, insomnia, poor sleep, dry skin, acne, blurry vision, sudden need to urinate, rash, stomach ache, swollen hands, knees, ankles, or feet, and, finally, flatulence. If you know what triggers allergic response, you are ahead of the game. If you are hypersensitive to certain foods, you simply take them out of your diet. There are hundreds of possible allergens, and it is impossible to list them all here.

Many people suffer from allergies to milk, eggs, wheat, and other grains. If you do not already know your limitations, start testing as soon as possible. Allergies are the first step to obesity and disease, as it all starts with diet.

To evaluate your daily life and habits, get an 8.5" x 11" notebook, and keep a journal. Recording what you eat and how you feel after eating it will help you to discover which foods make you feel weak and ill and will lead to pain and suffering if you continue to consume them.

Realizing that you can control your health is very empowering, is it not?

## Most Common Allergy-Causing Foods

| | | |
|---|---|---|
| Cereals | Oats | Butter |
| Caffeine/Coffee | Cashews | Crab/Lobster |
| Melons | Rye | Cheese |
| Buckwheat | Fish | Bacon/Pork |
| Dressings | Pecans | Sodium Nitrate |
| Peanuts | Wheat | Cottage Cheese |
| Corn | Shrimp | Chicken |
| Mayonnaise | Walnuts | Cottonseed Oil |
| Almonds | Milk | Ice Cream |
| Noodles *(Pasta)* | MSG | Luncheon Meats |
| Strawberries | Sausage | Corn Oil |
| Alcohol and Spirits | Palm Oil | Sodas |
| Processed Sodium | Eggs | |

## Foods That Help Detoxify

| | |
|---|---|
| Broccoli | Tangerines |
| Grapefruit | Romaine Lettuce |
| Cherries | Coconut |
| Cauliflower | Oranges |
| Bell Peppers | Green Onions |
| Artichokes | Dark Leafy Veggies |
| Garlic | Lemons |
| Cayenne | Asparagus |
| Collard Greens | Carrots |
| White and Red Onion | Limes |
| Cabbage | Blueberries |
| Brussels Sprouts | Raspberries |

Buy organic foods when possible. However, if you must choose between eating an allergy-producing food or eating a non-organic healthy food, go for the non-organic. Non-organic is always preferable to allergy-producing foods.

## Mucus Forming Foods

When cooked foods are eaten, large amounts of mucus are secreted. Foods that are particularly likely to produce mucus include:

| | |
|---|---|
| Meats | Pastas |
| Pastries | Cheese |
| White Flour Products | Candy |
| Processed Foods | Milk Products |
| Condiments and Salt | |

All processed foods leave us with mucus, and the body reacts by trying both to flush itself of waste and to protect itself by swelling.

Mucus is formed as a defense mechanism as the body resists toxicity. The mucus forming foods listed are often referred to as "Glue Foods." Nature provides mucus as a protective coating which surrounds gluey material in order to keep the intestinal membranes from absorbing toxic substances. When cooked foods are eaten, the T Cells, which are central to our immune function, increase the gastrointestinal tissue density *(swelling)* while increasing mucus production to keep toxins from leaching directly into the blood stream.

When toxins do leach into our blood, it is called "leaky gut syndrome," and can stimulate numerous forms of illness, including all types of arthritis, fibromyalgia, and diabetes, etc.

CHAPTER 12

# Food Combining
# and Beyond

## Meat Proteins Do Not Combine with Starches

Leading the list of our worst illness-producing habits is combining meat proteins with starches. If you are familiar with the trials of digestion, you know that the combination of meat proteins and starch simply cannot be easily digested.

I am frequently asked, "What about meat and potatoes, hamburgers, sub sandwiches, pizza with meat, macaroni and cheese, hot dogs, etc?"

Let's look at the "All-American Hamburger." The meat is a protein, and the bun is a starch. It takes large amounts of digestive acid to break down a "compost bin" of competing opposites. When we consume acids and alkalis in the same meal, they neutralize each other, creating a chemistry lab technician's nightmare. Not surprisingly, the same is true in the stomach. Your system tries to sort it all out, but slow, flatulent digestion is the result. When our meals do not digest properly, they rot in the gut from beginning to end, like foods in a compost bin. A healthy body with a good, balanced diet seldom has flatulence. John Tilden, M.D. says, "Nature never produced a sandwich."

Plant-based proteins such as avocados and legumes will safely combine with all starchy vegetables and grains.

## Fruits Do Not Combine with Starches

Fruits and whole-fruit sugars require little digestion since they begin digesting readily because of their natural enzymes. Processed starches, such as breads, require the most digestive time. From the time we put food into our mouths, our bodies start reacting to what we are eating. If we eat a mish-mash of foods, the body is confused.

The rule of thumb when eating fruit is: Eat only fruit when eating fruit. Do not combine fruits with other foods. This, of course, means we do not eat raisin bran, preserves on toast, bananas in our cereal, carrots in slaw with raisins, etc. It is a lot to think about, but food choices are important decisions.

## Melons Do Not Combine with Vegetables or Other Foods

Melons combine with no other food, as they are a near-perfect food. They literally require no digestion in the stomach and quickly pass into the intestines. If melons are left in the stomach at 104 degrees while waiting with another, slower-digesting food, the melon begins to rot/ferment.

Put a piece of melon outside in the sun at 80-90 degrees, and you will see it rot before your eyes. If you eat melons with any other foods, you are setting yourself up for digestive disturbance and stomach problems later. Is it any wonder that so many people are bothered by melons? They do not know this important fact and routinely make easily correctable errors when eating melons. There is no exception to the rule: Eat melons alone, or leave them alone.

**High-Acid Fruit Does Not Combine with Low-Acid Fruit**

If you understand pH, you know that all fruit has a pH of less than 7.0 and is, therefore, acidic. Citrus fruits are highly acidic in the area of 2.2 on the pH scale. Bananas are in the vicinity of 4.9, which makes them much less acidic than citrus, although the difference between them is only 2.7 points. On the pH scale, that is a huge difference. The best choice when eating fruit is to eat it alone, and do not combine types of fruits.

**High-Acid Fruit**

| | |
|---|---|
| Grapefruit | Cranberries |
| Lemons | Currants |
| Limes | Gooseberries |
| Tangerines | Loganberries |
| Kumquats | Strawberries |
| Pineapples | |

**Less-Acid Fruits**

This underappreciated group of fruits deserves more recognition than it sometimes receives.

| | |
|---|---|
| Apricots | Papayas |
| Apples | Blackberries |
| Pears | Blueberries |
| Cherries | Figs |
| Nectarines | Grapes |
| Peaches | Guavas |
| Plums | Mulberries |
| Mangoes | Raspberries |

Do not combine bananas, carob, dates, pineapples, or plantains with the fruits listed above.

## Dried Fruits

Dried fruit is popular, but the addition of sulfur as a preservative and denatured enzymes cause many people trouble. If this is true for you, be wary of dried figs, peaches, pineapples, prunes, raisins, apples, and apricots.

Keep in mind that what is on your plate today determines your health tomorrow and into the future.

# CHAPTER 13

# Testing

## Lab Test

Get a weight loss blood panel from your doctor to learn what your potential hurdles will be. Your test will show what factors in your blood are responsible for gaining weight. Be sure your panel includes tests for all the following:

Estradiol
DHEA
Free Testosterone
C-Reactive Protein
Progesterone
Glucose
Homocysteine
TSH
Triglycerides

Kidney Function
LDL Cholesterol
HDL Cholesterol
Total Cholesterol
Liver Function
Free T4
Free T3
Complete Blood Cell Count

In addition, your doctor should check for High Blood Pressure and order an EKG.

## Candida Yeast Test

Try this fast and free saliva test. At night before you go to bed, put ¾ cup of water into a clear glass, and place it on your night stand. In the morning when you awake, before you put anything in your mouth, put some saliva in your glass of water.

Wait 10 minutes and look at the side of the glass. If the saliva has strings hanging in it or if it sinks to the bottom of the glass, there is Candida yeast present in your body. That could cause weight gain.

**Barnes Thyroid Test**

To perform this test you will need a basal thermometer, a clock, and a note pad close to your bed to use upon waking in the morning.

Before bed, set your digital thermometer to "start" or your analog thermometer to 95 degrees. Upon waking, do not get up or expend any energy before placing the thermometer against the skin of your armpit. Allow 10 minutes to measure your temperature, and note your temperature on a pad.

Repeat this test for five consecutive days.

Your temperature should be in the range of 97.4 to 98.5.

If your temperature is higher than 98.5, you may be hyperthyroid *(overactive)*.

If it is lower than 97.4, you may be hypothyroid *(underactive)*.

With a little knowledge in your hands, you can be far more successful in your quest to lose weight.

CHAPTER 14

# Other Weight Loss Methods

**Herbal Products**

An extract from a West African plant called Irvingia has been shown to help maintain healthy body weight. However, herbal products advertised as "metabolism enhancers" or "fat blockers" usually purchased over the counter at a health foods store do not do anything more than make users sick.

**Fasting**

Fasting has long been employed to help the body with weight loss and detoxification. It is an ideal weight loss booster. The recommended way to incorporate fasting into your weight loss plan is to choose one day a week to abstain from eating. The day to miss meals is your choice. If, for example, skipping Sunday is less stressful for you than another day, skip Sunday. Try to choose a day that can be consistent for you.

**Alternative Treatments**

For some people, body wrapping has been shown to produce results. Acupuncture is another age-old technique which helps some people. Some swear by hypnosis, but, in reality, anything that can be accomplished by hypnosis can be achieved by using your own willpower.

## Commercial Diet-Based Programs

Support programs that aid dieters in keeping their word to themselves require on-going monthly payments for counseling and/or meals delivered to your house. This is a multi-billion dollar industry, but the public continues to grow more and more overweight.

## Exercise-Based Programs

Fitness centers, often called gyms or health clubs, are fee-based programs as well, and may be paid weekly, monthly, or yearly. Here you find personal trainers, but in the end, it requires your determination, sweat, and persistence to make a difference. Most people attend a club only a few times then lose interest. These businesses bank on this behavior. Working out may not take off weight as quickly as diet restriction, but in the long term, it is better for you.

## Pre-Packaged Meal Plans

Your body needs real, whole, fresh foods, not canned, frozen, or processed foods. Whole raw foods are best since they digest themselves.

## Meal Replacement

Meal replacement can be good for a couple of days, a week, or even a month, but not for the long term. You should work with a natural health counselor to build a personal program.

## Surgery

In addition to being dangerous and expensive, surgery exemplifies the classic placebo effect. Weight loss surgery does not do anything but remove parts. Weight loss after surgery is the result of the mandatory diet restrictions and exercise requirements that follow the surgery. Do not waste your time on this dead end method. Lap Band and Gastric Bypass surgeries claim to heal diabetes, but they do not. Those who have had bariatric surgery and follow the recommended dietary guidelines notice that diabetes vanishes.

Diabetes is not changed by altering the digestive plumbing, but it is affected by diet change and exercise. If one loses weight after surgery, it occurs because the person followed the mandatory, but often not followed, post-operation recommendations. When one does not follow those recommendations, no amount of surgery will aid weight loss. The post-bariatric surgery demands are immense, but are often ignored. Among many others, well-known people including Chris Christie and Carney Wilson have had weight loss surgery and have not lost weight.

To lose weight after weight-loss surgery, patients must adhere to a program of eating smaller portions, drinking more water, eating fresh fruit and vegetables, eliminating all junk food, and adding daily exercise. You may be wondering how following the previous guidelines would not result in weight loss. The plain truth is that gastric bypass alone does nothing. Without diet and exercise, gastric bypass is a pointless exercise in unnecessary elective surgery. The fact that post-surgery diet change and exercise controls diabetes, and the surgical plumbing change does nothing is embarrassing, to say the least, to the "Big Diabetes" industry.

## Lifestyle Modification Program

No matter how detailed your plans for building a house, until you take the actual steps of construction, you still have no house. Similarly, weight loss requires a series of actions, including diet change and exercise. Whatever avenue we take, diet and lifestyle changes are absolutely necessary. Otherwise, we are only kidding ourselves.

## Medications

Don't expect medications to work for long without changing your diet and lifestyle, drinking plenty of water, and getting regular exercise.

Stimulants will work until you "blow a gasket," perhaps in your heart or maybe in your brain. Is that the avenue you want to pursue? I hope not. It is up to you to decide what course of action is best for you and to embrace it fully. Choose life and habit changes, and you will win the battle and live to tell others about your journey.

# Testimonials

**Rebecca**

I met Dr. Hakeem when he was consulting with my husband. My husband had been experiencing headaches daily for the past three years.

Dr. Hakeem reviewed some of the foods my husband was consuming to determine which ones were causing the headaches. My husband followed Dr. Hakeem's suggestions and eliminated certain foods. Soon his headaches stopped.

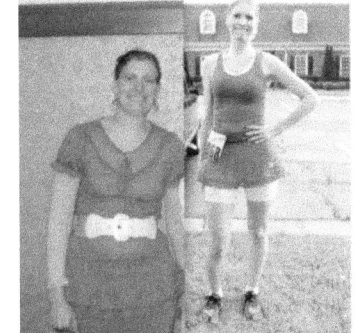

I followed the same information Dr. Hakeem used to counsel my husband on his food selections. By just adding a regular exercise program, I dropped from 180 pounds to 135 pounds. It only took me four months.

**Amanda**

I told Dr. Hakeem that I wanted to lose six pounds. I am 5'2" and weigh 125 pounds. Dr. Hakeem smiled and said, "Where?" Dr. Hakeem suggested I use digestive enzymes. I followed his advice, and in nine days, I lost six pounds.

**Gloria**

Dr. Hakeem informed me that it would be best to start a program to lose weight in the fall. I am 5'5" and 180 pounds. After following his directions, I am a "star student," having lost 25 pounds! I am very pleased with my progress.

**Carrie**

I started my weight loss program with Dr. Hakeem by doing whole body purification. When I started, I weighed 214 pounds. I am 5'4", and am now 175 pounds. I have not felt this good in five years.

# Testimonials

## Carol

Dr. Hakeem knows the method to the madness of healthy weight loss. I have been learning about my food sensitivities and healing on a cellular level. Anyone can use Dr. Hakeem's principles for healthy living to lose weight through lifestyle changes that really work. I have lost forty pounds, but even more importantly, I am healing my body on the cellular level.

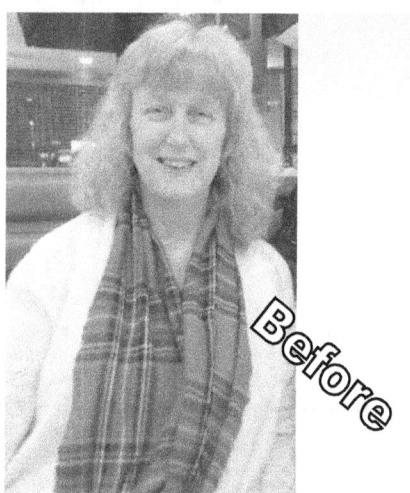
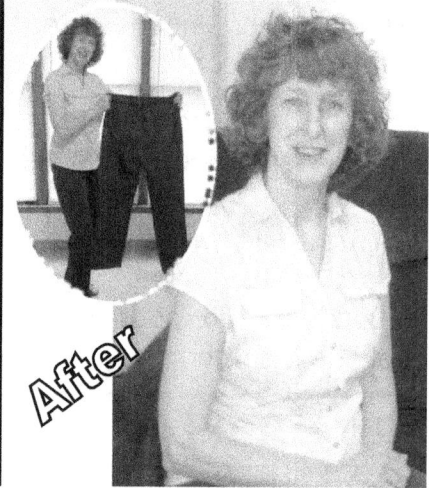

## Marvin

My wife told me about Dr. Hakeem. She told me that he has a great weight loss approach. I asked him how much weight I could lose, and he told me it was up to me, based on my determinations and drive. That was 4 ½ months ago, and I am down by 56 pounds and now weigh 175 pounds at 5'8". I am as good as I was in high school.

## George

When I started my weight loss program with Dr. Hakeem, I was on a lot of medication and weighed 210 pounds. I am now down to one medication and am only 182 pounds. Not bad for being 5'10".

# *A note from me to you.*

Don't be in a hurry to lose weight, you should lose between two and three pounds a week. Getting healthy is a process and no one expects you to be able to do it overnight. It takes time to make life changing alterations. We can have a good relationship between our food and health. **You can do it.**


I wish you the best.

Dr. Abdul Hakeem

Watch for my upcoming book on,

**Whole Body Purification Program.**

For release notifications please send your e-mail address to:

drhakeem1@gmail.com

I want to think all of my friends and clients for purchasing,

## Steps To Take Before Starting A Weight Loss Program.

*(Soon available in Audio book)*

Each reviewer of my book will receive a free 30 minutes complimentary consultation *(a $195 value)*.

**I'm also available to do health workshops for churches and non-profit organizations at a reduce price.**

The diet you have today,
may determine your health in the future.

SO, ENJOY LIFE.

**Dr. Abdul Hakeem,** Ph.D., N.D., N.C., Bio-C.P. is in private practice in Greensboro, N.C., providing holistic health care. The counseling of my clients is centered around teaching them how to build excellent health from a holistic approach using Western, Ayurvedic and Chinese disciplines. I assess the clients health through an examination of blood pressure, and pulse, body temperature, finger nails, tongue, facial skin, body type, body chemistry, age, weight, body type exercises, and the condition of their immune system.

1. How to develop a positive attitude.
2. How to use diet, body type exercises, massage, stress management, sunlight, water, meditation, internal cleansing, whole body purification program, organic supplements, herbal formulas, and spices properly.

By using these programs you may be able to reduce or reverse weight and poor health conditions. These programs look at the physical, mental, emotional and spiritual well-being of the individual.

For more information go to my web-site at:
www.thecenterfornaturalliving.com

www.ingramcontent.com/pod-product-compliance
Lightning Source LLC
Chambersburg PA
CBHW070821290526
45795CB00002B/792

* 9 7 8 1 5 1 1 7 8 1 6 5 7 *